Finding Food For Survival

A Guide to Trapping and Obtaining Food

Prepping and Survival Series

M. Usman

Mendon Cottage Books

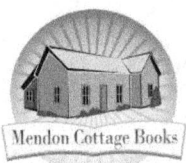

JD-Biz Publishing

Disclaimer

The information is this book is provided for informational purposes only. It is not intended to be used and medical advice or a substitute for proper medical treatment by a qualified health care provider. The information is believed to be accurate as presented based on research by the author.

The contents have not been evaluated by the U.S. Food and Drug Administration or any other Government or Health Organization and the contents in this book are not to be used to treat cure or prevent disease.

The author or publisher is not responsible for the use or safety of any diet, procedure or treatment mentioned in this book. The author or publisher is not responsible for errors or omissions that may exist.

Warning

The Book is for informational purposes only and before taking on any diet, treatment or medical procedure, it is recommended to consult with your primary health care provider.

Our books are available at
1. Amazon.com
2. Barnes and Noble
3. Itunes
4. Kobo
5. Smashwords
6. Google Play Books

Table of Contents

Preface

Food is the primary necessity of life. Although it is clear that lack of availability of food will not kill you instantly, it will deprive you of the energy you require to get yourself out of any survival situation.

Desperation makes people lean towards some insane choices and our help here is to provide you with sane options of your food sources in different kinds of survival terrains. Be it wilderness, desert, or snow, food is one of the key assets to survival. This book aims at guiding you to the best food sources these areas can provide you with.

Plants can be your savior as you do not have to catch them, but there is a catch here as well, since you have to identify the plants that are safe for you. Don't worry, we will try to cover this part extensively.

Not all of us are trained hunters. This book gives you some tips on how to set proper traps to catch some protein in the wild. Remember, this is not for fun, it is for survival and only the fittest can survive. Just follow our advice and always be prepared for emergencies by keeping a good knowledge of the whereabouts of your adventure zones.

Chapter 1 – Introduction

In a survival scenario, food is one of the three most pressing issues that you have to face, along with water and finding a place to rest. Food is what drives you, both emotionally and physically, and to survive from these terrible scenarios you need food to reenergize yourself. Remember the times when you had an empty stomach and were forced to perform a task? Not fun, is it? Even worse is when you are out there in the wilderness where you need all your focus and energy. Lack of food will hinder your path to finding help.

In a survival situation you have to take advantage of everything that you can find to eat. Most wild terrains are full of natural food, ranging from plants to animals. The food sources you can exploit are determined by the habitat you are in. You have to vary your diet to make sure you get the appropriate amounts of proteins, fats, carbohydrates and vitamins. We will discuss some of the different terrains where you might have the misfortune to stumble and lose your path. We shall try and provide you with a basic overview along with specifics on various terrains.

Meat and fish are good sources of protein and fat and provide virtually everything a long-term survivor might require. At the first part of a survival scenario, plants are the most fitting diet as they are easily available and contain the necessary nutrients for human consumption.

Chapter 2 - Relying on the Greens

In the wilderness when you do not have your stock of reserve foods with you, plants can offer you nutrition for survival. Plants though can be really tough to manage and it is absolutely essential that extreme caution must be taken before their consumption. There are many poisonous plants out there that can make the situation quite bad for your if digested. Poison hemlocks, for instance, gets mistaken for wild carrots and kill off a number of people.

Let us initiate with a few instructions on picking out the wild plants that are safe for you.

Keep the following in mind when collecting wild plants for food:

- Plants growing near homes and vehicles can be contaminated by the poison that we create. Hence we should avoid picking them from close to these sites.

- Some plants develop extremely dangerous fungal toxins, therefore spoiled fruit and vegetables are a bad idea. No matter how desperate the situation, look for cleaner parts.

- Plants growing in contaminated water are contaminated themselves. You should boil them before eating.

- Plants of the same species may have different toxic content because of genetic or environmental factors. An example of this is the plant life of the common chokecherry. Some chokecherry plants have high amounts of deadly cyanide compounds while others have low concentrations. Avoid any leaves, weeds, or seeds with an almond like scent, a common characteristic of the cyanide compounds.

- Some edible wild plants, such as acorns are bitter. Boiling them will usually remove these bitter properties and make them better for utilization.

- The key thing to remember is that you should never ever eat a wild mushroom. The mushrooms consumed may not show any sign of damage at first, but within a couple of days your nervous system will breakdown. Do not take that chance with your life.

Universal Edibility Test

It is not humanly possible to be able to learn about all the plant species that exist. It would be foolish to think that you have a command over this knowledge. To remove this obstacle, researchers have provided us with a unique universal edibility test. There are several components for this test. Let us initiate this discussion.

Separate - Not all parts of the plants are edible. So the first task that we have to do is to separate the leaves, roots, stems, buds, and flowers. Then you should check the parts for worms and other insects. Confirmation of worms is a good sign that it's rotting. Discard the plant in this scenario.

Contact - After the separation of the components, you need to perform a contact test. If your skin cannot bear the plant, your stomach is bound to suffer as well. Crush the part of a plant and rub it on your wrists. You have to wait for eight hours now. Do not continue with the plant if it irritates you. A burning sensation, redness and bumps are all terrible signs. During the waiting period you can only take water.

Cook – Plants can have their toxins removed if cooked properly. Get ready to boil the plant initially and then taste it. Keep it on your lips for about three minutes. The same steps are to be done if you are testing the plant raw. If the food shows no negative reaction on your lips, continue with testing. Withdraw otherwise.

Taste - The plants that clear the cooking test are to be moved forwards for tasting. Hold the plant with your tongue and do not swallow. Wait for five to fifteen minutes, and if you experience any unpleasant sensation spit it out. Bad taste does not means that the plant is toxic, what you are looking for is burning sensation or tingling on your tongue.

Chew - If tasting survives, you may start chewing the plant. Thoroughly chew the plant for around five minutes. Swallow only if you feel that you are not experiencing any negative reactions.

Swallow - What you have at the end of your ordeal is a very soggy piece of plant in your mouth. But now we have to show the real patience as after this mushy swallowing, you are not allowed to eat anything for eight hours more. After this waiting period if you feel that your condition is turning terrible, induce vomiting and use lots of water.

Chow – Finally the last step is chewing down the same part of the plant. Prepare it similar to the first three steps. Wait another eight hours and as always you may take water, but you have to refrain from eating anything else.

We leave you with a few important notices:

- Never eat plants with thorns.

- Avoid plants with shiny leaves.

- Mushrooms are not worth the risk.

- Plants with white or yellow berries should be avoided.

- Avoid plants with seeds inside a pod.

- If it tastes bitter, spit it out.

Chapter 3 - Plant Options

There are various options and choices among plant selections as the terrain changes.

Temperate Zone Plants

- Asparagus

- Blackberries

- Amaranth

- Blueberries

- Plantain

- Nettle

- Daylily

- Sassafras

- Thistle

- Water lily and lotus

- Pokeweed

- Wood sorrel

- Cattail

- Chestnut

- Chicory

- Dandelion

- Strawberries

- Oaks

- Prickly pear cactus

- Wild onion and garlic

- Wild rose

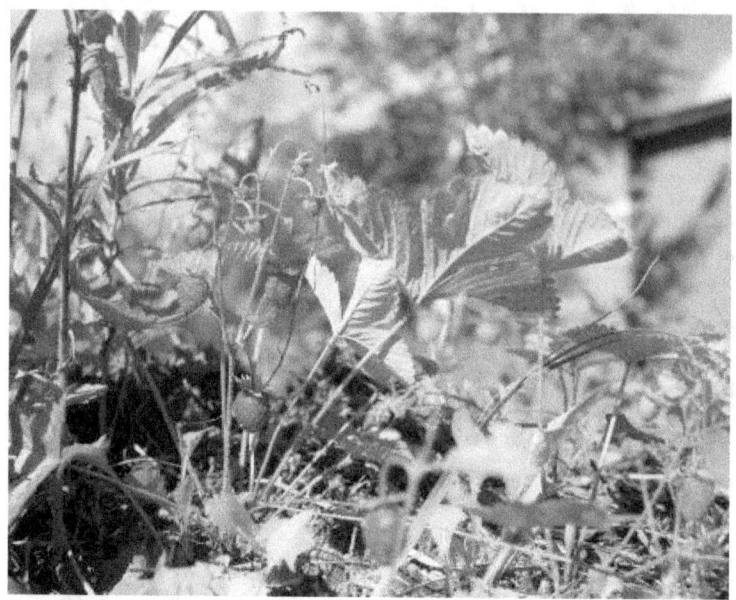

Tropical Zone Food Plants

- Bamboo

- Bananas

- Coconut

- Breadfruit

- Sugarcane

- Mango

- Cashew nut

- Papaya

- Palms

- Taro

Desert Zone Food Plants

- Date Palm

- Agave

- Cactus

- Desert amaranth

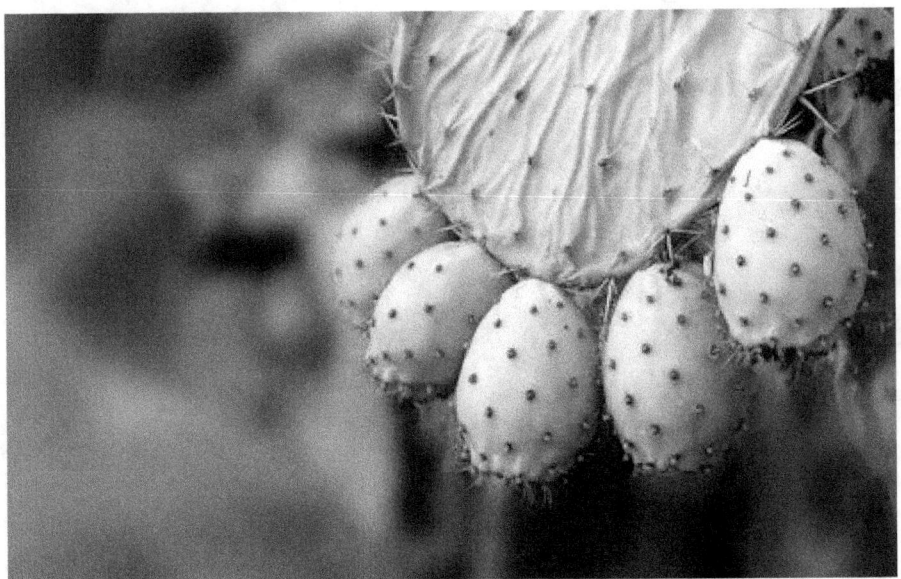

North African Plantation

Conifers

The inner bark of conifers, known as the cambium layer, is filled with calories and sugar. Most evergreen and cone-bearing trees provide us with this luxury. Yew, identified by the red berries, has to be kept at a distance from oneself and should not be consumed.

Grasses

All grasses are edible. The leaves can be chewed and the juices swallowed, but you should spit out the indigestible parts. The root corm which is the part where the base of the leaves meet the roots should be roasted. It can be eaten like a potato.

Oaks

All acorns and the nuts produced by oak trees can be leached of their bitter tannic acids and eaten. They are filled with protein, fats, and calories. The acorns can be placed into several changes of boiling water to remove the tannins.

Chapter 4 - Desert Survival

Food spoils very quickly in the desert and any food material, once opened, should be eaten at once or kept covered for later use. Remember that this later use has to be within a very short span. Flies will appear suddenly and settle on your uncovered food and will start ruining your dish. The most important thing that you need to keep in mind is that when in a desert, you really should not eat more than you need to recover your energy. In the heat of the desert, eating more will increase your metabolic heat and cause more water loss in your body. Since finding and replenishing water is the main problem in deserts, you need to avoid this situation. Keep your focus on the fruits and vegetables that you can find and try to lay off the proteins. You will need water to digest the food that you consume so make sure that you eat lots of food with moisture.

Animals that you can find in these regions are insects, reptiles, and a few specially adapted animals for specific regions. For instance, you have the Australian bandicoot, the fennec fox of north Africa, the jack rabbit of North America and the hedgehog from Gobi. All of these animals have large ears that act as cooling aids. Other animals that hide in the sands include geckos, lizards and snakes.

The deserts have their own share of curious animals that have properties that enable them to survive in these rough conditions. The Sahara has gerbils and gerboas; the Middle East has caracals and hyenas, and in the region of Kalahari there are squirrels that can use their tails for shade against the raging sun. There are gazelles that manage to absorb all the moisture for their needs from the sap of the leaves. The feathers of the birds give them insulation against the heat and they can breed long distances apart from the water sources. The road runner from Arizona is a famous example.

Reptiles are a good protein source and relatively simpler to catch. You should always seek to eat them after cooking, but in a troubled situation, you can eat them raw. Raw flesh has another drawback, as it may transmit parasites, but because reptiles are cold-blooded they are free from these harmful parasites and do not carry the blood diseases of the warm-blooded animals. Quite obviously you need to avoid the hazardous reptiles like snakes and alligators as they are more likely to make you their prey.

As hard as it might be for most of us to imagine, ants, grubs, and grasshoppers can be consumed. One fine strategy to get over our natural reluctance to eating bugs is to toss them into a stew with other more tasty ingredients. Insects constitute of the most abundant life-form on earth. Their advantage is that they are easily caught. Insects give us 65 to 80 percent of rich protein, which is a huge amount when compared to the 20 percent we obtain from beef. This fact makes insects an important, if not overly appealing, food source. Insects to avoid include all adults that sting, bite and are hairy or brightly colored. You would also do well for yourself if you can avoid spiders and the famous common disease carriers that are ticks and mosquitoes.

Tips for Finding Food in the Desert

1.   If water is not available, do not eat.

2.   You should have plenty of water before you exhaust yourself in looking for food; you ought to conserve your sweat so that your bodily fluids last longer.

3.   AVOID plants with milky sap.

4.   AVOID all red beans.

5.   AVOID bitter or soapy taste.

6.   AVOID spines, fine hairs and thorns.

7.   AVOID dill, carrot, parsnip and parsley like foliage.

8.   AVOID "almond" scent in woody parts and leaves.

9.   AVOID grain heads that have black spurs or are pink and purple.

10.   AVOID three-leaved growth pattern.

11.   If possible, boil plants that are questionable.

12.   Use the "Universal Edibility Test" if you doubt a plant is poisonous.

13.   Unless you're an expert hunter, don't hunt; use trapping instead since it has less effort involved.

Some Common Desert Edible Plants

1.   Abal: Its fresh flowers can be eaten in spring.

2.   Acacia: The young leaves, pods and flowers of Acacia are edible raw and are even better when cooked.

3.   Agave: Its flowers and flower buds are safe to eat, but just to be certain you should always boil them before eating.

4.   Cactus.

5.   Date palm: Its fruit is edible fresh but is very bitter if eaten before it is ripe.

6.   Desert amaranth: All parts are suitable for eating, but some may have spines that have to be removed before consumption.

7.   Desert raisin

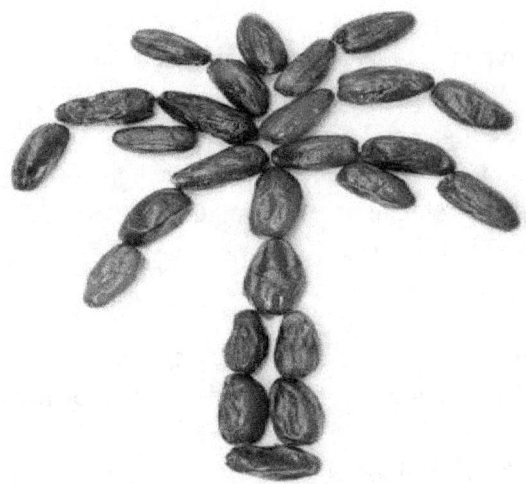

Chapter 5 - Survival at Sea

Almost all sea life is not only fit for human consumption, but is rather an excellent source of nutrients that are essential for human survival. Seafood is high in both minerals and vitamins, thus becoming a luxury for people.

Tips for Finding Food in the Open Seas

- Conserve energy.

- Try fishing and spear fishing at night because it's the easiest.

- Poisonous fish are more commonly a found on the reefs, in several coastal regions.

- Plankton is another healthy option for humans to procure, nutritious and easy to catch are some of its surplus advantages.

- A golden tip is that you should not eat food until you have water. Of course it is not possible to starve yourself; eating less is the hidden wisdom.

- Baits have to be used. Convenient baits are the smaller fish that you catch; their organs can also be used for this purpose.

If a fishing kit is available, the task of fishing becomes a jolly good task. The rafts and the shadow it brings can attract the smaller schools of fish towards itself. These fish can be eaten or used as bait for larger fish. Another thing that attracts fish is light, so a flashlight or the reflection of the moon can be used. Now it can be very dangerous if the line is secured to either you or the raft is because a larger fish may cause more harm than good.

Seabirds have proven to be a useful food source, which may be more easily caught than fish. Birds can be shot, grabbed or baited by hooks. Once you kill the birds they should be skinned to get rid of the oil glands. It is always better to cook the bird but drastic conditions can also call for raw consumption. The flesh should be eaten or preserved immediately after cleaning. The unused parts can always be used as bait.

Birds might land on your raft to rest or circle you in search of food. This brings your food right at the door and that's a great chance to catch them by hand, a net, or you can spear them. Remember there are no fixed rules to catch them and you can always improvise!

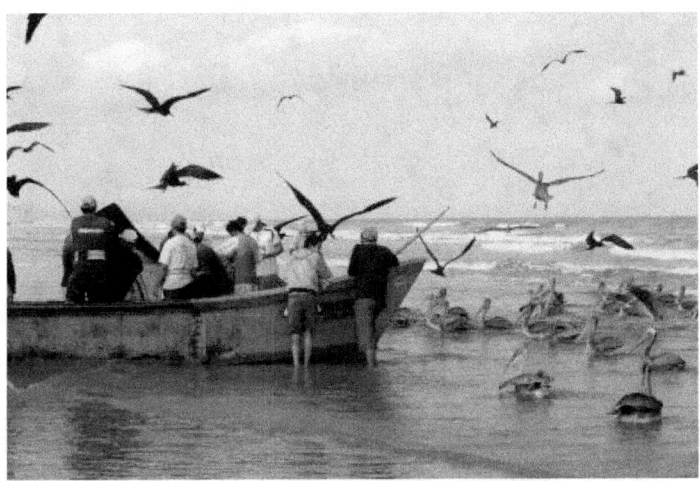

Plankton is very nutritious. Whales (whale, sharks, and manta rays) feed on large quantities of plankton, therefore all areas hosting those marine animals will be filled with plankton. Plankton will often be found on the surface at night, and it goes much deeper during the day. Any type of net with very small holes dragged behind a raft will work well.

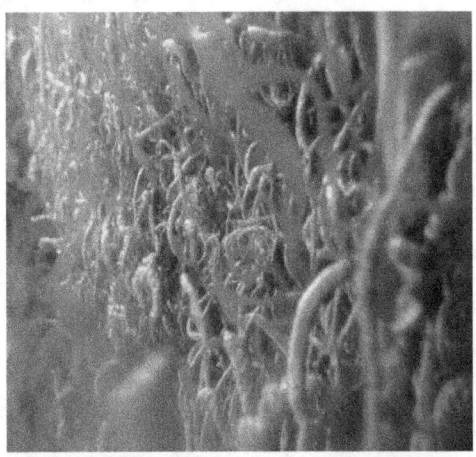

Seaweed of various types is found on most oceans. Most seaweed are edible, however some green or blue algae found in freshwater pools can be highly poisonous. Most type of seaweeds are found in coastal areas either drifting or still attached to rocks. Seaweed that has been washed onto the beaches and dried out cannot be consumed as it is hard to eat raw. Dry the seaweed in the sun or if you can conjure up fire, that will be even better. Below are some types of seaweeds;

- Dulse

- Green seaweed

- Irish moss

- Kelp

- Laver

- Mojaban

- Sugar wrack

All sea life must be cleaned perfectly and eaten as soon as possible otherwise the food will be wasted, as it cannot be conserved.

Chapter 6 - Setting Traps and Snares

The one thing that is even more important than learning how to set the traps is learning where to place them. Position your traps and snares where there is proof that animals pass through. You must determine if it is a "run" or a "trail." There is a difference between a run and a trail. A trail will show you signs of use by several groups of animals and will be quite different. A run on the other hand, is smaller and less distinct and will only contain signs of one particular animal. Location of the trap matters. Animals have bedding areas and feeding areas with trails leading and tracing location. You have to recognize all these areas to make certain that your efforts are not getting wasted.

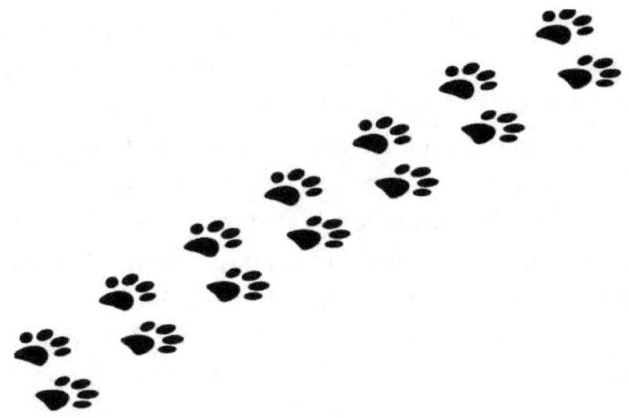

Act like a ninja. It is very important, not to create a disturbance that will alarm the animal and cause it to avoid the trap. Remember that they may have keener senses than you have. Therefore, if you must dig, remove all fresh dirt near the trap. Animals will by nature and strong senses avoid a danger trap. To avoid this situation prepare and construct the trap elsewhere and remove signs of human touch to the trap. In case you disturb the local plantation the animal will become suspicious. Freshly cut vegetables are a bad idea in setting a trap. Freshly cut vegetation will "bleed" sap that has an odor the prey will be able to easily grasp that smell and the alarm is raised.

All human senses should be removed from around the trap that you set. You cannot deceive mammals with appearances alone; their sense of smell is very sharp. Even the slightest human scent on a trap will alarm the prey and cause it to avoid the area. It is exceedingly difficult to completely remove the human scents from around a trap, but what you can achieve fairly easily is that you can mask that smell. Use the fluid from the gall and urine bladders of successfully trapped animals. Human urine is not advisable. A good alternative is mud obtained from an area with plenty of rotting vegetation. Use it to coat your hands when handling the trap and to coat the trap when setting it. Animals only get alarmed by the presence of the fire itself; smoke does not alarm them so it can be used to mask the human scents as well.

Traps placed on a trail or run should use channelization. For this channelization, you should aim for a funnel-shaped barrier. It should be extending from the sides of the trail in the direction of the trap, with the narrowest part positioned closest to the trap. Channelization should be subtle to avoid alerting the prey. As the animal gets to the trap, it should have no alternative directions to move into, hence making the trap a more likely success. The barriers do not have to be brick walls; you only have to make it inconvenient for the animal to go over or escape between the trap. For excellent above par results, the channelization should minimize the trail's width to just slightly wider than the targeted prey. Keep this restriction as far back from the trap as the length of the body of the animal and then it should start to widen up towards the mouth of the funnel.

Use of Bait

Baiting a trap increases your chances of catching an animal. Success with a trap without using any bait solely relies upon its location. A baited trap can actually draw animals to it. The bait should always be something the animal recognizes. However, it should also not be so readily available in the immediate area that the animal can get it close by and end up ignoring your trap. For example, baiting a trap with corn in the middle of a corn field would not be likely to work. Likewise, if corn is not known widely in the locality, its bait in the trap may engage an animal's curiosity and keep it alerted while it ponders the strange attractive food. Baits that work well on small mammals are peanut butter and salty foods. When using such baits, scatter bits of it around the trap to give the prey a chance to sample it and develop a liking for it. The animal will then slowly overcome some of its fear and get accustomed to the surroundings before it gets to the trap and will fall into a false sense of security. Hit and trial methodology is a given here, the animals do not have a preference list. You will have to observe and deduce with experiments as to what baits which specific animals respond.

Trap and Snare Construction

Traps and snares crush, choke, hang, or entangle the prey. I know it sounds mean, but we are not doing this for fun, it's an emergency and the survival of the fittest applies. If you do not hunt and your condition weakens, you can turn into the prey. A single trap or snare will commonly incorporate two or more of these principles. The struggling victim, the force of gravity, or a bent sapling's tension, provides the power. The heart of any trap or snare is the set off. When planning a trap, ask yourself how it should impact the animal, the power providing source, and what deciding the most efficient trigger.

Types of Traps

A simple snare is a noose placed above a trail attached to a firm tree. If the noose is a type of cordage placed upright on the trail, use small sticks or some grass roots to hold it up. An excellent object for holding up the noose is the filaments from the spider webs. You have to ensure that the noose is large enough to easily pass over the neck of the animal and as it moves forward, the noose can then tighten itself. The noose gets tighter as the animals struggle. This trap is best done with a wire and it does not result in the killing of the animal, it simply traps it.

Drag Noose

On the run of an animal use a drag noose. Place forked ticks on the sides of the run and lay a sturdy cross member diagonally to their position. Tie the rope to the cross member and hang it carefully at a height that should be above the animal's head. As the noose tightens around the neck of the animal it pulls the cross member from the placed sticks and forces them to get dragged along the line. The surrounding plants quickly catch the cross member and the animal becomes tangled.

Twitch-Up Snare

A simple twitch-up snare consists of two forked sticks, each with a long and a short leg. First bend the twitch-up and mark the trail directly under that line. Next you need to push the longer leg of one of the sticks forcefully into the ground at the marked point. Make sure that the cut on the short leg of this stick is parallel to the base or the ground. Tightly tie the longer leg of the remaining stick to a piece of cordage, make sure that it is firmly secured to the twitch-up. Next cut the short leg so that it catches on the short leg of the other forked stick. After completing the attachment, extend a noose on top of the trail. The trap is then set by bending the twitch-up and engaging the shorter legs of the sticks. The forks are pulled apart as an animal gets struck, causing the prey to get hanged.

Bottle Trap

A bottle trap is a simple trap for animals like mice. The dimensions of the hole have to be 30 to 45 centimeters deep, wider at the bottom and narrower at the top. Make sure that the top of the hole is as small as possible. Place a piece of wood over the hole with small stones under it to fill it up to a height of 2.5 to 5 centimeters above the ground. The animal will hide under the cover in order to evade the lurking danger but will ultimately fall into its own doom. The slope prevents any chances of the animal climbing back. Just be cautious of any lurking snakes.

Squirrel Pole

A squirrel pole is a large pole placed against a tree in areas where there are a lot of squirrels located. One noose will not do the trick on this occasion and you have to place several nooses on the top and sides, so that the squirrels moving up and down will eventually get trapped in one of them. Position the nooses so that they are 5 to 6 centimeters wide, approximately 2.5 centimeters apart from the pole. The top and bottom wire positions of the rope should be around 45 centimeters apart to ensure that the pole will prevent the squirrel from getting its feet on the ground. Otherwise the squirrel will end up chewing through the wire. Being naturally curious, after an initial waiting period, they will experiment with the pole and will be caught.

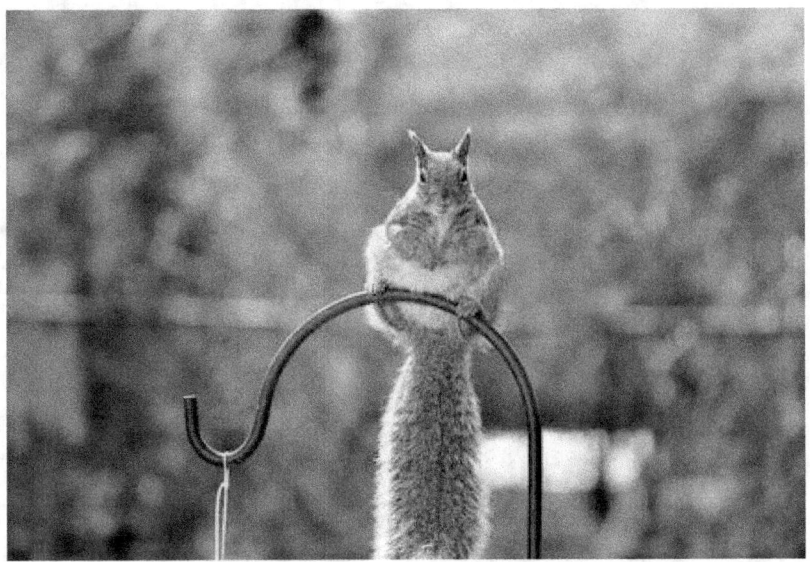

Ojibwa Bird Pole

The Ojibwa bird pole has been used by the Native Americans for centuries. This trap is for areas that are more open rather than an area dense with trees, and the best areas are near the feeding, dusting or watering holes. Firstly, cut a pole roughly 2 meters long and clear off the plants. Do not use resinous wood such as pine. Sharpen the upper end and then make an opening of a small diameter of 5 to 7.5 centimeters down. The next step is to cut a small stick 10 to 15 centimeters long and shape one end so that it will almost fit into the hole. This is known as the perch. Plant the long pole in the ground with the pointed end up. Tie a small weight, roughly equal to the weight of the prey, to a length of rope. Spread one end of the cordage through the hole and tie a slip noose that completely covers the perch. Next, tie a single overhand knot in the cordage and place the perch next to the hole. Next, let the cordage to slip through the hole so that the overhand knot rests against the pole and the top of the perch. Meanwhile, the tension of the knot will hold the perch in the right place. As the bird lands, the perch will fall and the noose will tighten around the feet of the prey.

Fish Traps

There are several methods to catch fish and a fish basket is one of these. You construct them by joining several sticks together with vines into a funnel shape. You can also use traps to catch fish, as they regularly get dragged upon the shore with the incoming tides. All you need to do is to pick a location at high tide and form the tricky trap at exact low tide.

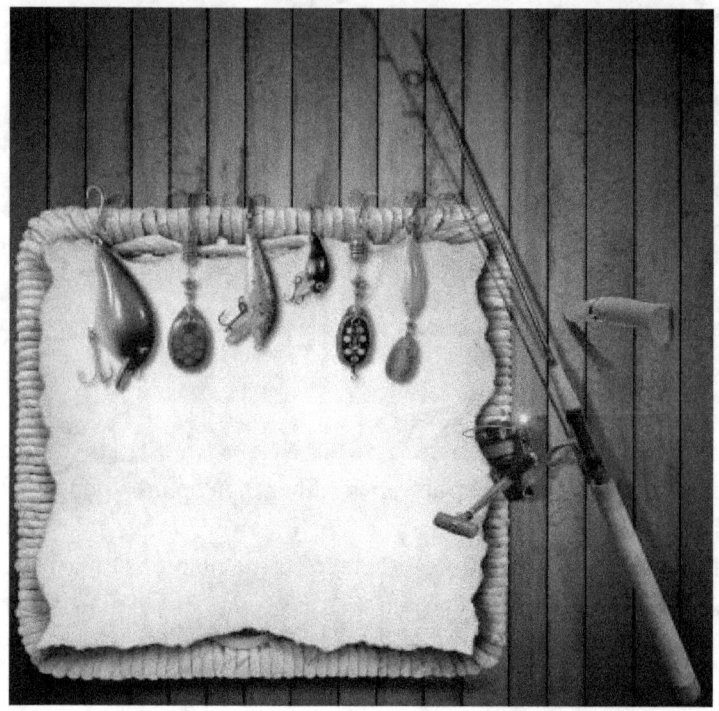

Chapter 7 - Conclusion

Food collection is a tricky process and not to mention a tedious one too. So make sure that you have all the essentials and only need to use the wild food as a last resort. Although some plants or plant parts are eatable raw, you must cook others to make them edible. Edible means that a plant or food will provide you with necessary nutrients. Many wild plants are edible, but barely delicious. Since we need to try and make the food we consume tastier we can try several techniques to make this happen. Methods used to improve the taste of plant food include boiling, leaching, and the most obvious cooking. Leaching is done by crushing the food by placing it in a strainer and immersing it in boiling water. Stuff like this can be really helpful too, so learn all this before your adventures, because no one knows when a calamity strikes.

Author Bio

Muhammad Usman is a distinguished medical graduate of Allama Iqbal medical college (AIMC). He is a professional writer who has been in the field for more than 4 years. During this time he has produced 10,000+ articles, blogs, and eBooks on various niches related to diseases, health, fitness, nutrition and well-being. He is a regular contributor to several journals related to medicine and surgery. He is the editor of several journals and newspapers.

Check out some of the other JD-Biz Publishing books

Gardening Series on Amazon

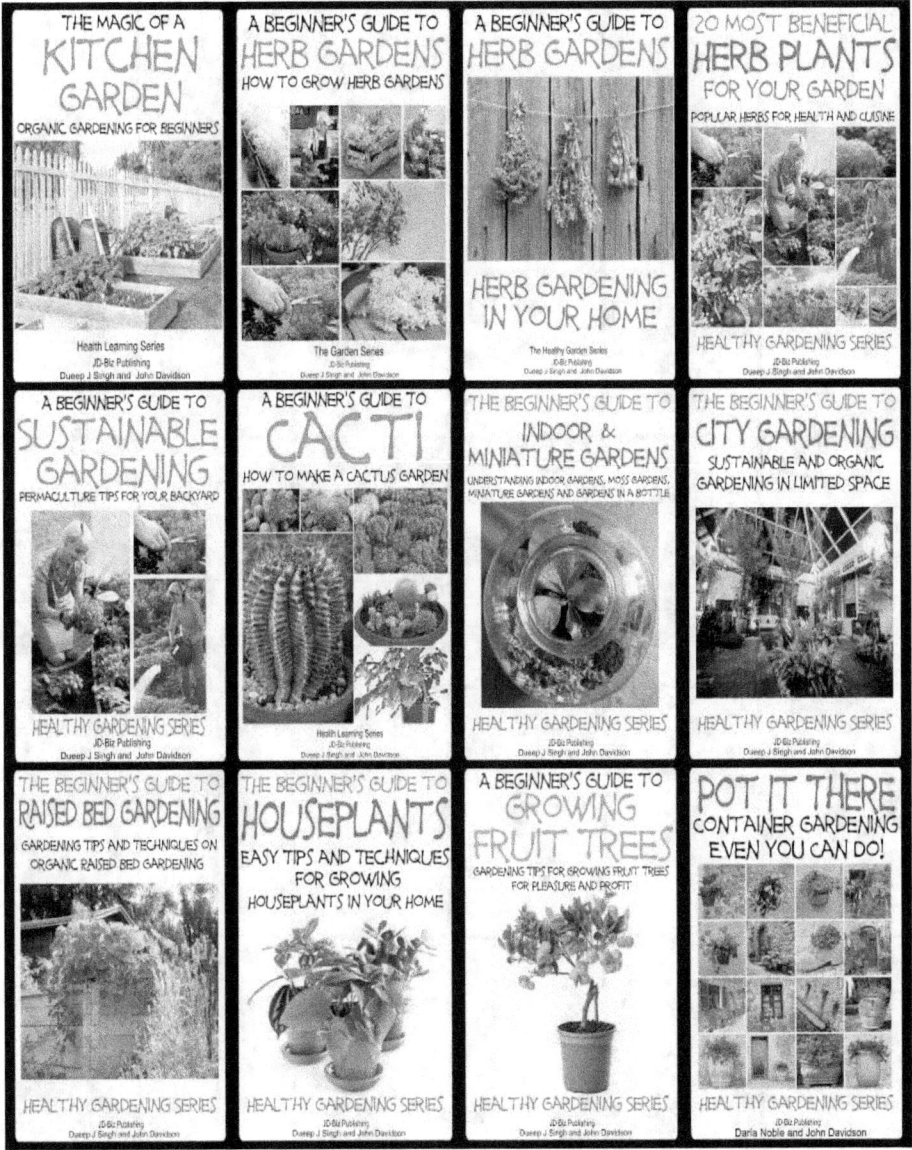

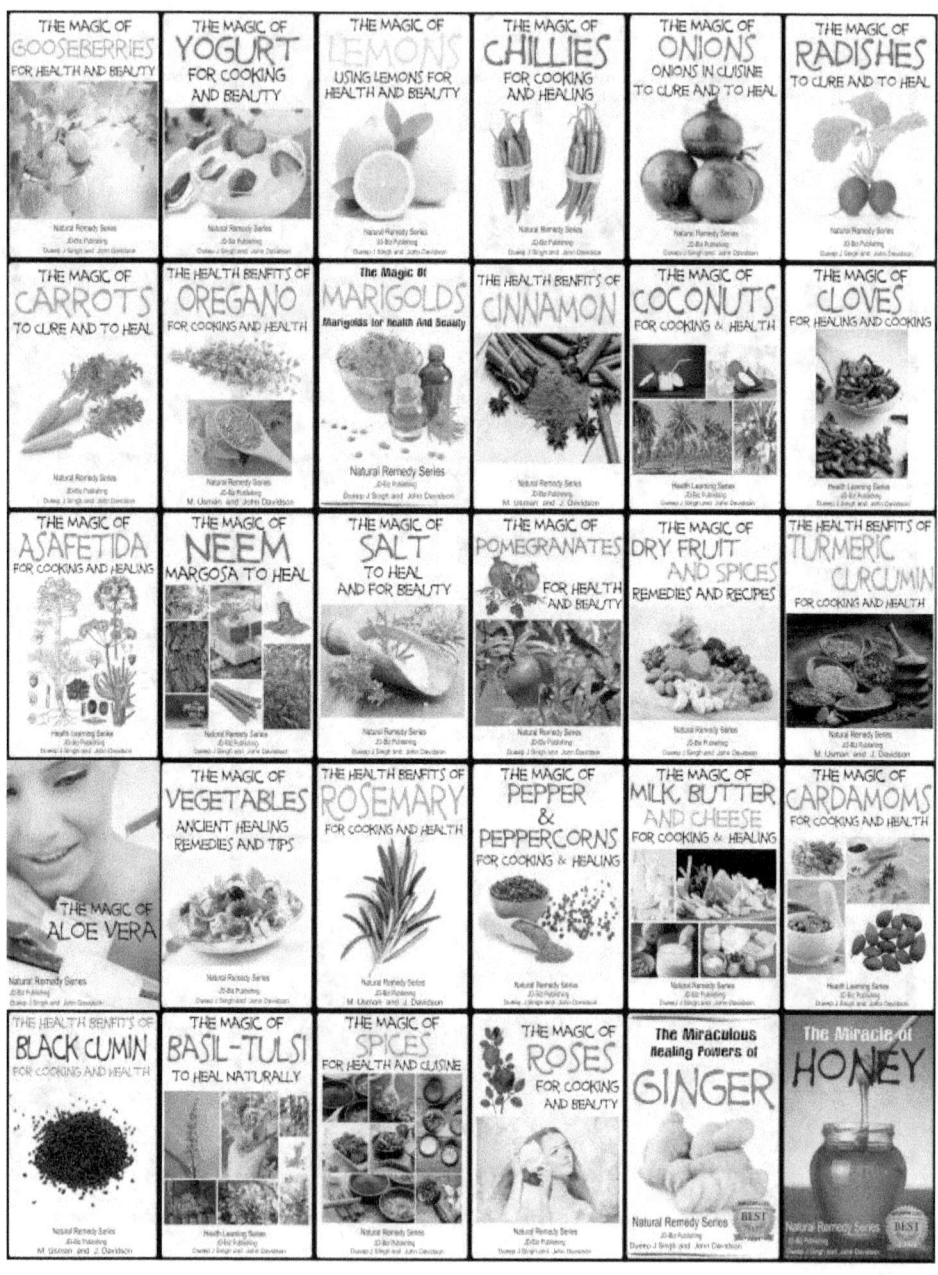

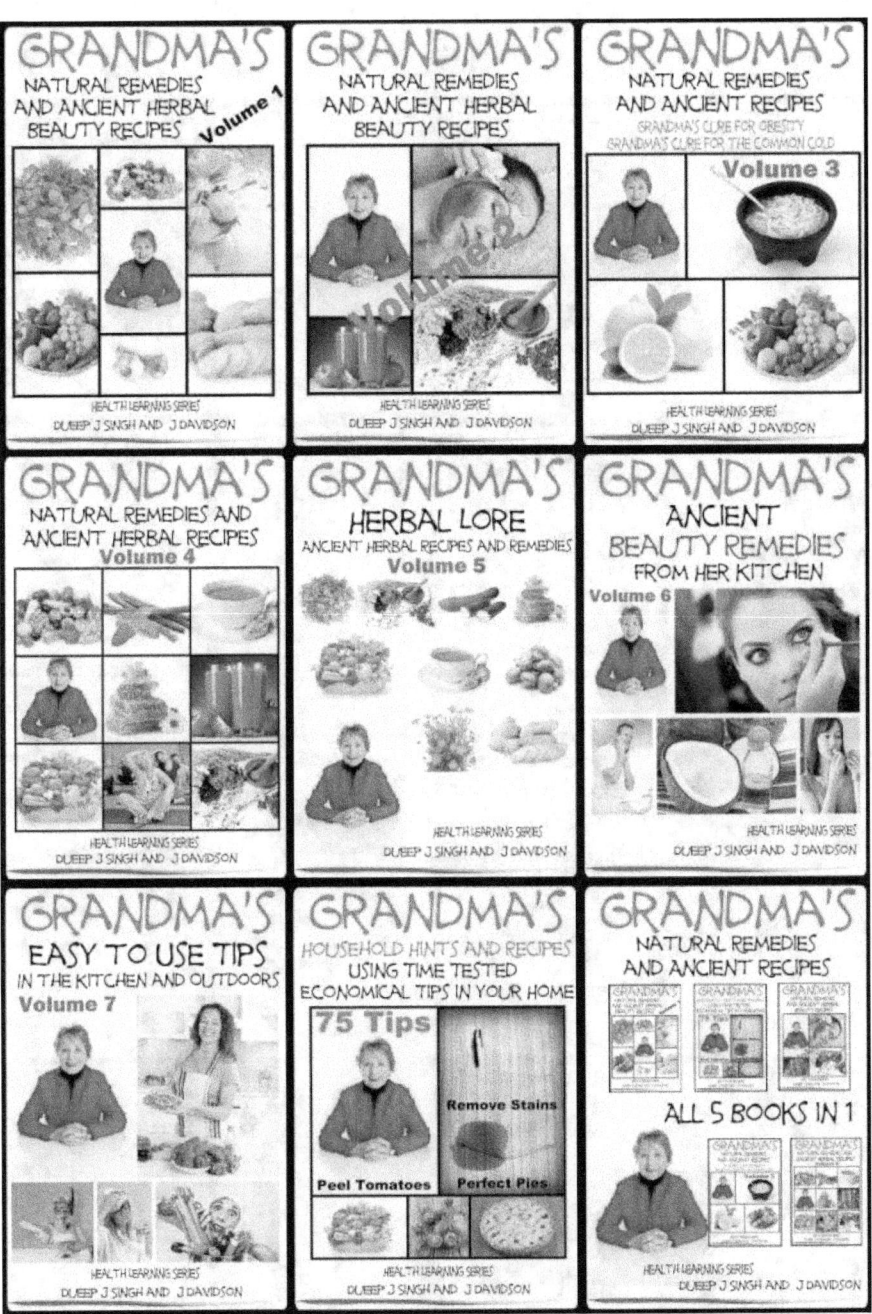

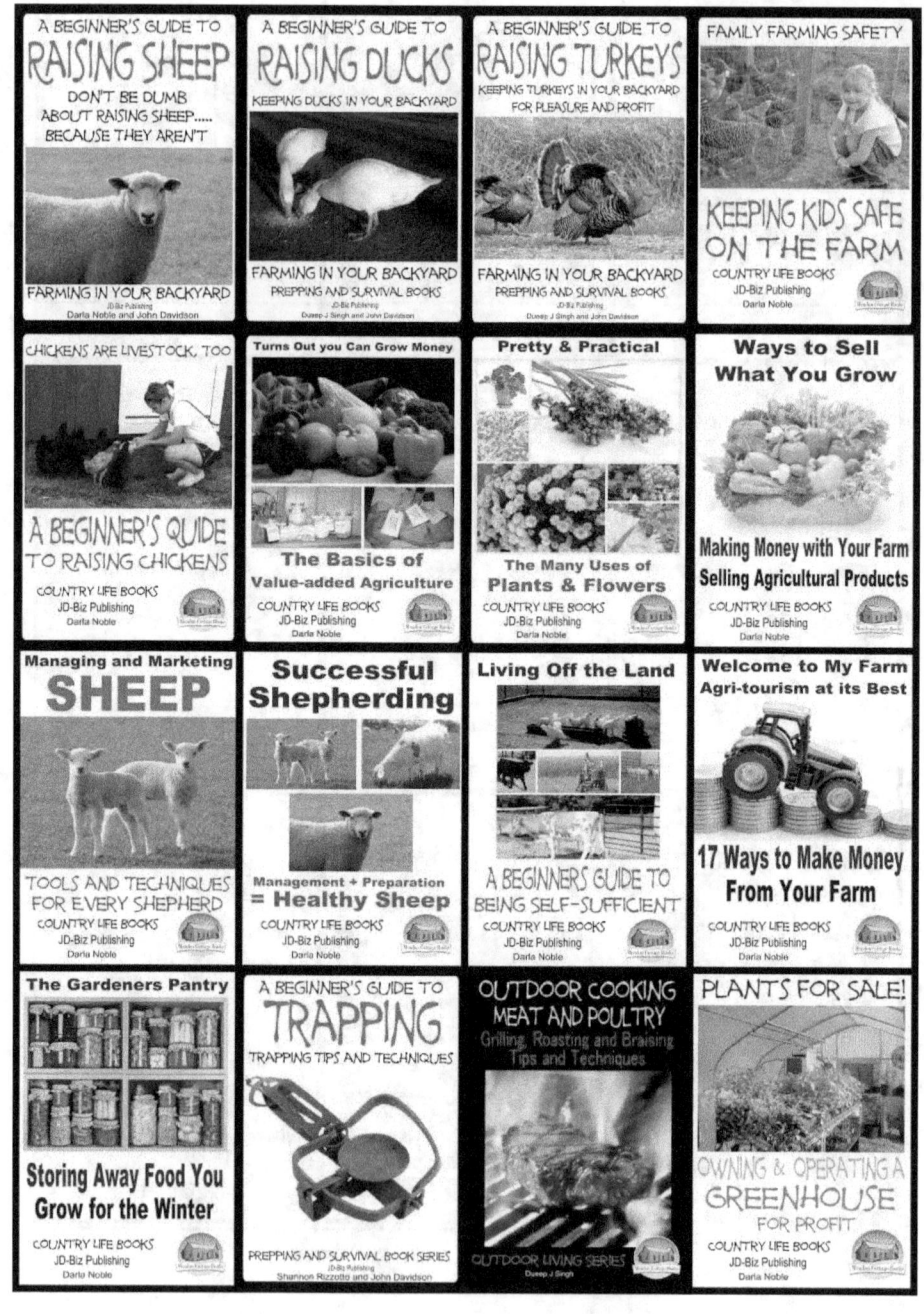

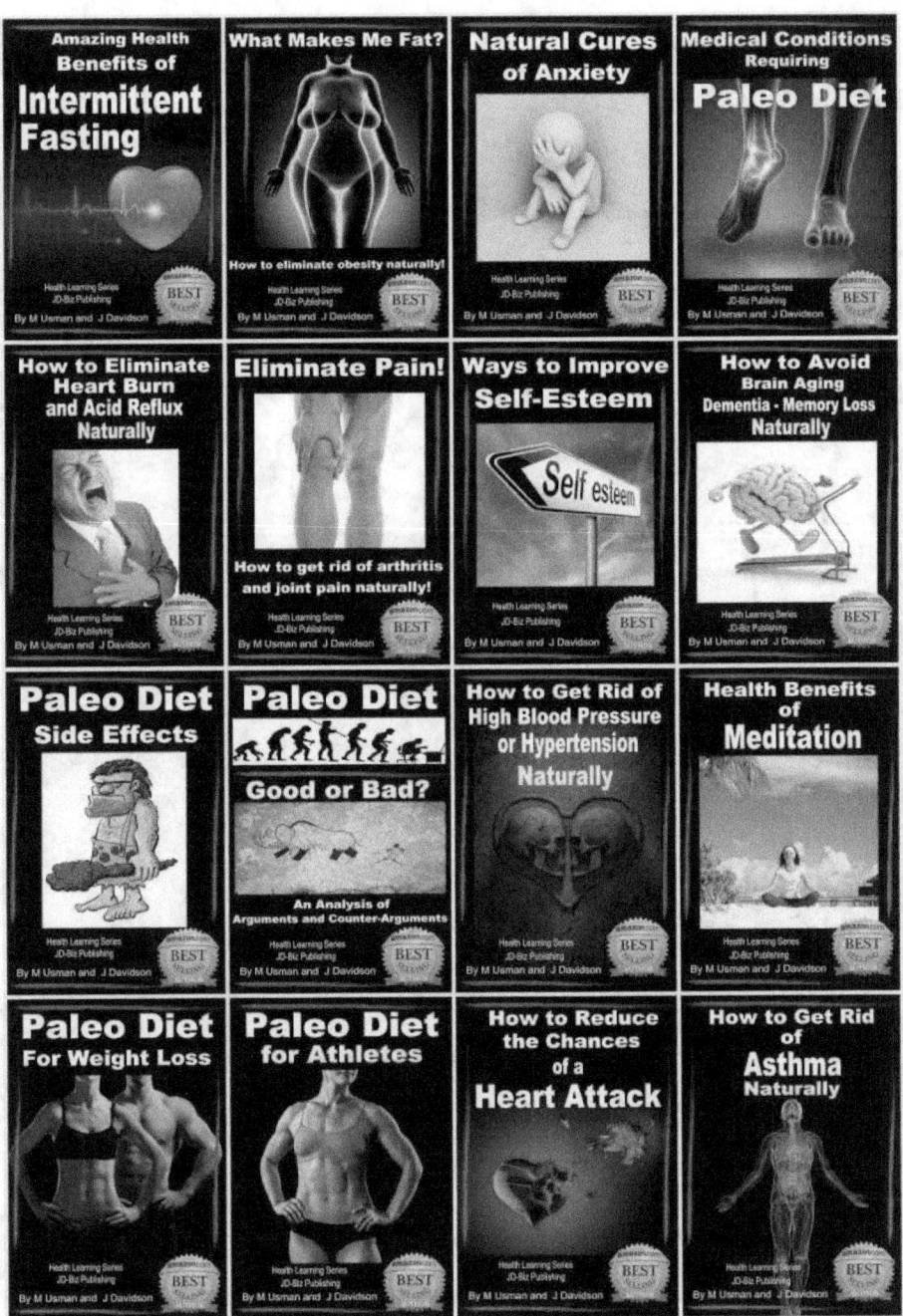

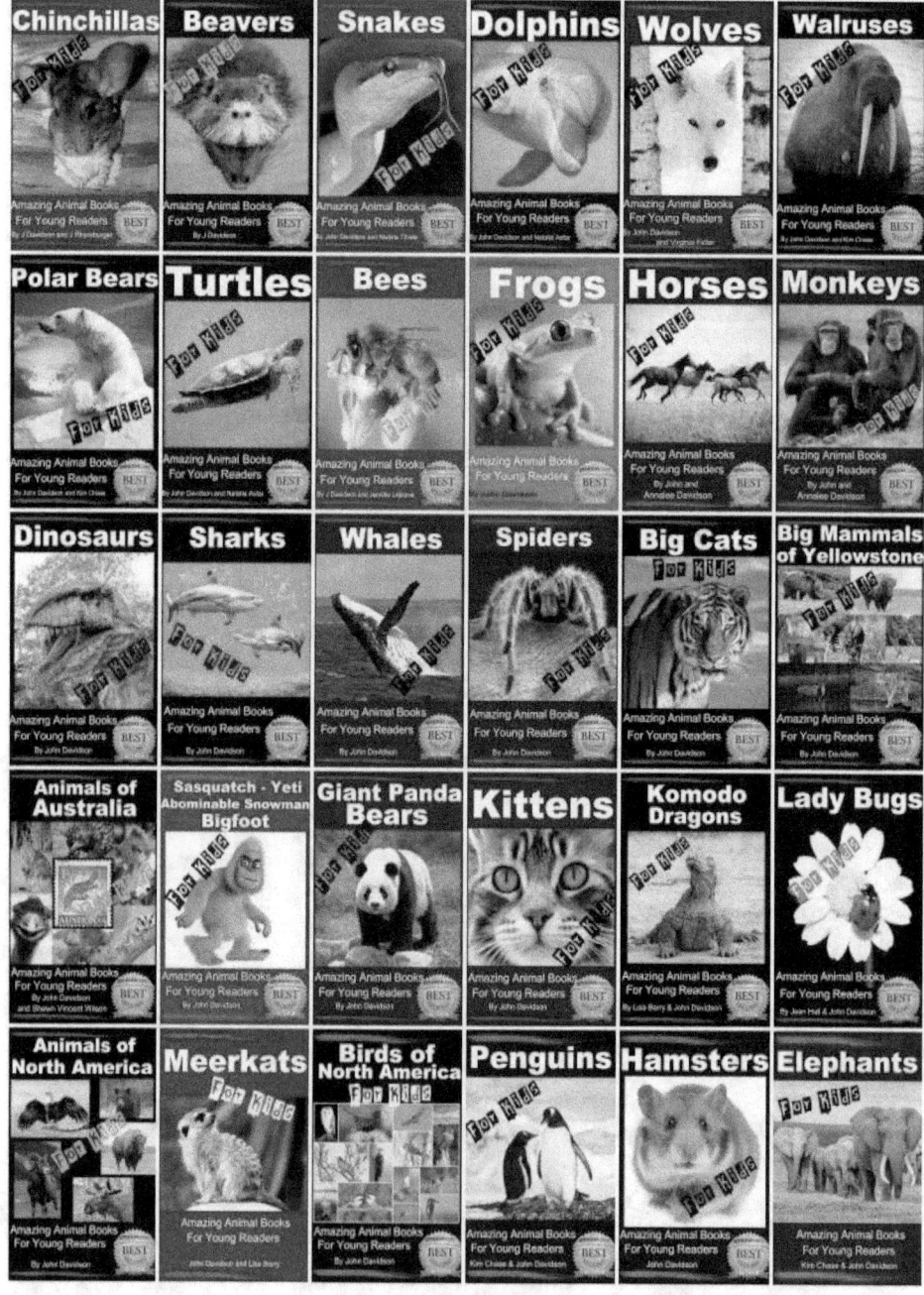

Learn To Draw Series

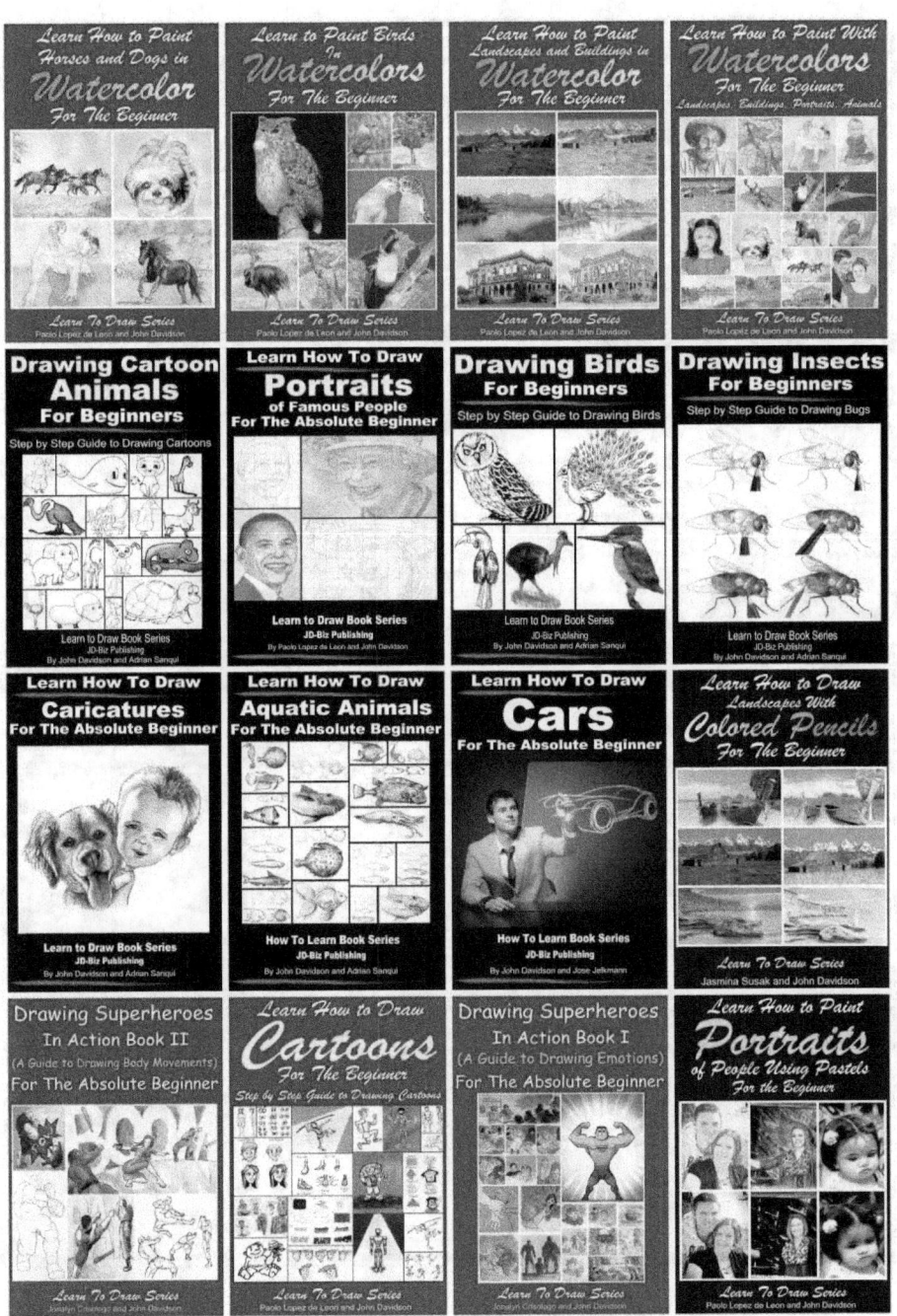

How to Build and Plan Books

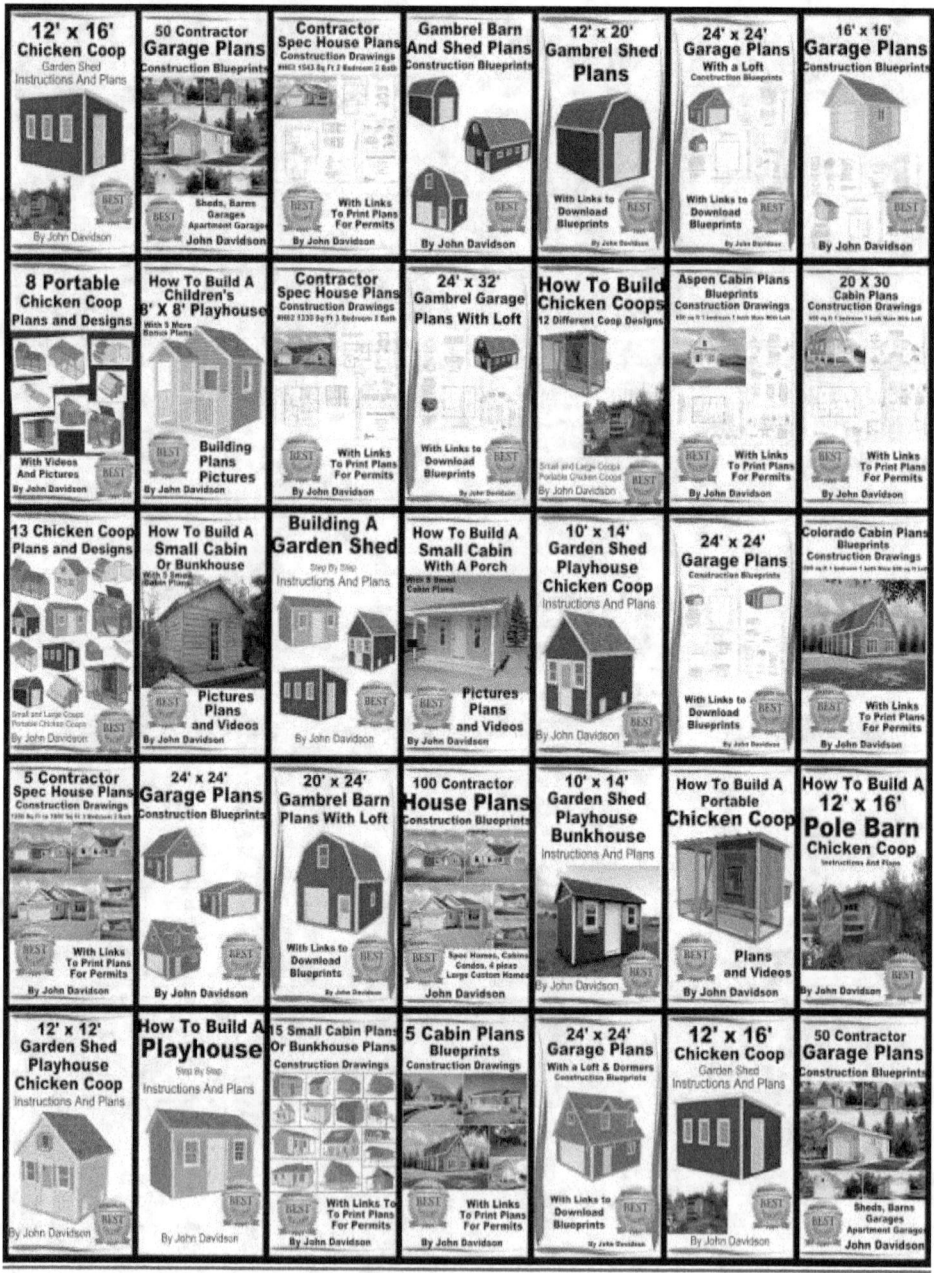

Entrepreneur Book Series

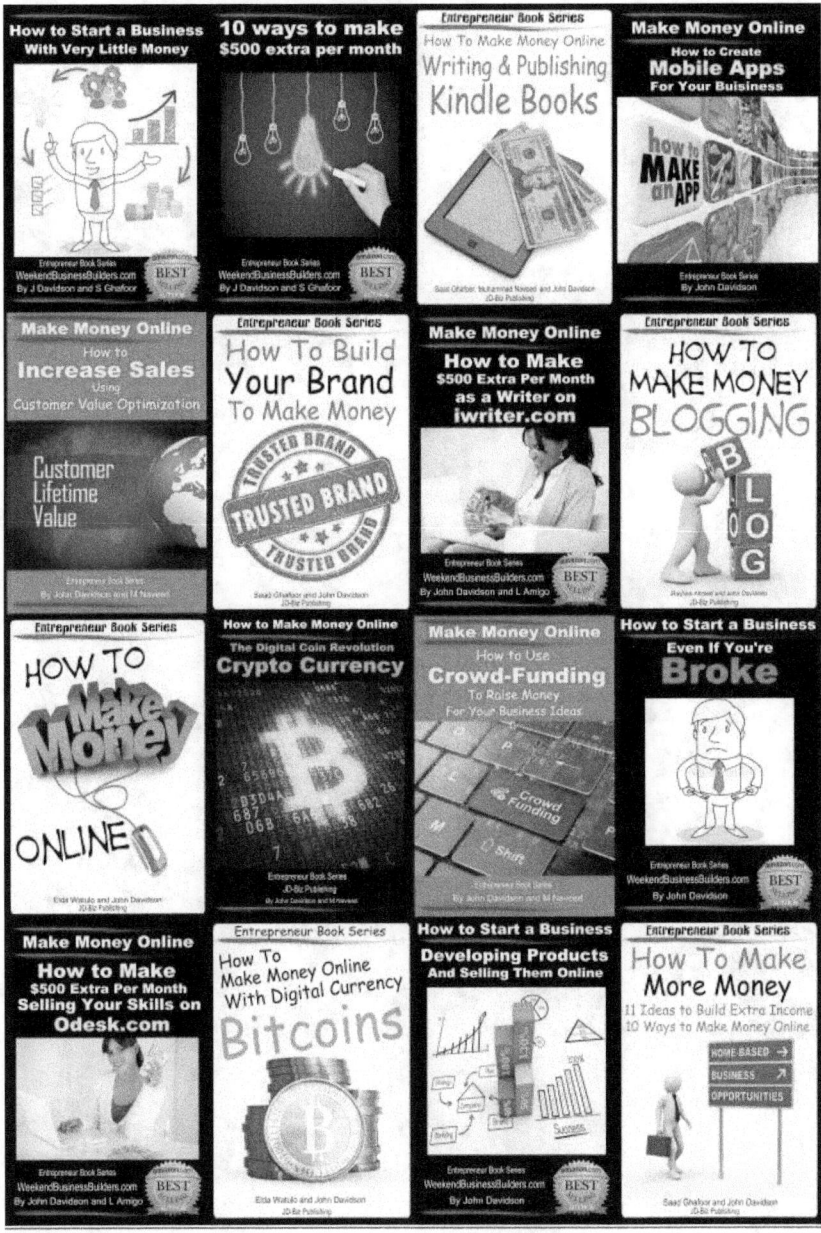

Our books are available at

1. Amazon.com

2. Barnes and Noble

3. Itunes

4. Kobo

5. Smashwords

6. Google Play Books

Publisher

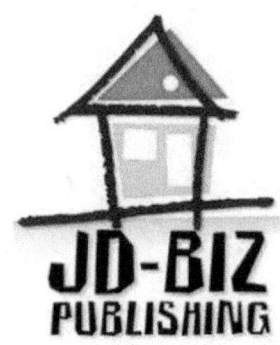

JD-Biz Corp

P O Box 374

Mendon, Utah 84325

http://www.jd-biz.com/

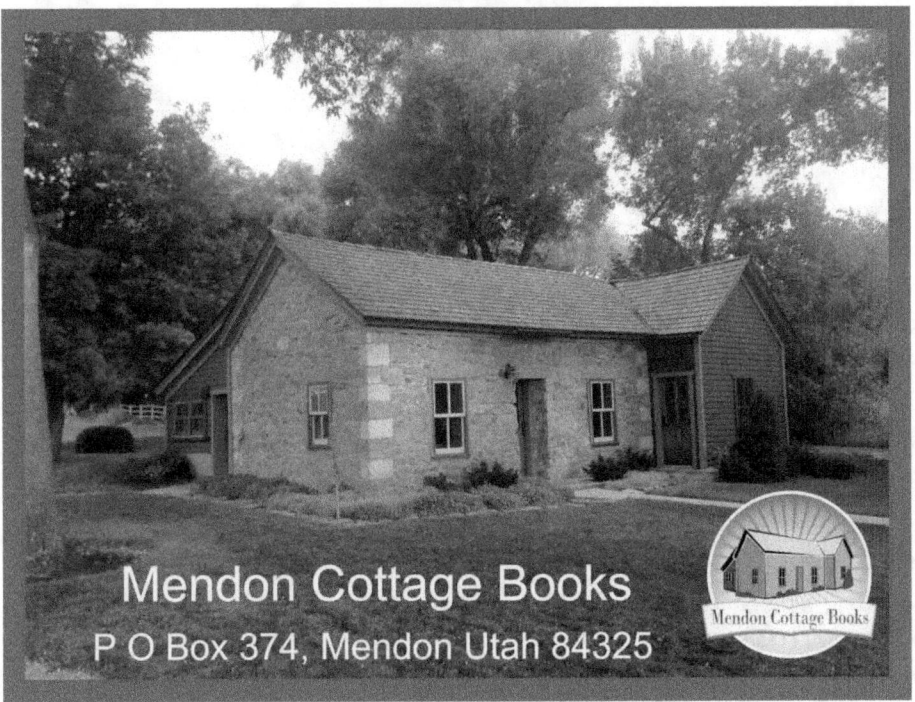

Mendon Cottage Books

P O Box 374, Mendon Utah 84325